How To Get An Ass:

A Detailed 6 Week Guide to a Bigger, More Toned, Gravity Defying Butt!

Leanne Wiese

© *2015*

Copyright/ Disclaimer Information

This book is not intended as a substitute for the medical advice of physicians. The reader should regularly consult a physician in matters relating to his/her health and particularly with respect to any symptoms that may require diagnosis or medical attention.

Table of Contents:

Foreword By: John Mayo

When my girlfriend asked me to write a forward for her book I was a little hesitant due to the specific subject matter. The topic of health & fitness is my true passion, but this particular book seemed a little bit too feminine and specific for my liking. Leanne assured me that I would approve of the book and after reading it for myself, I must admit that I do. As a man I had never really taken women seriously when I'd hear them commenting on men's asses, I had always thought that it was only men that cared about the shape of a woman's behind, but I guess it's a two way street!

Leanne is a true fitness fanatic. She is competitive, strong, focused and determined and as her boyfriend I have no problem saying that she has a great bum. She is a master when it comes to exercising in a way that really works her lower body, causing her bum to lift and creating fantastic shape. It's really no secret that men are attracted to women with nice asses, it's just in our nature. The workouts featured in this book are sure to give you the ass that you've always wanted.

Leanne is a certified personal trainer and creating workout programs is what she does best. She personal trains out of a gym that is strictly for women and her female clients have all seen results after being trained by her for only a few months. Leanne has taught me many of the exercises in this book and she has put me through nearly every single one of the workouts. This book receives my stamp of approval and I'm not just saying that because I'm dating the author. See for yourself, try the program, challenge yourself and get the ass you've always wanted!

Introduction:

Are you ready to get the ass of your dreams? Do you want to lift your booty up in a way that seems to defy gravity? It's no secret that men find a woman's bum to be a critical feature in determining her attractiveness. I'm not trying to degrade women; I'm just stating facts. Now ladies, I'm going to be honest with you, getting a toned butt with that natural perk and lift is a difficult thing to do. It requires discipline, focus, exercise and a proper diet. I will provide you with everything you need to know in the following pages. We will discuss dieting advice, the best exercises for getting a lifted butt, an in-depth 6-week workout plan and there will be 4 fantastic fitness tips dispersed throughout the book.

This isn't going to happen overnight. Unless you are one of the lucky few of us with fantastic ass genetics, getting the ass of your dreams is going to be a lot of hard work. As a side note to all those abovementioned ladies with lucky genetics, be wary; your amazing butt is not going to last forever without proper maintenance and if you've never really had to work for a killer booty then you probably don't truly appreciate it like someone who has. This complacency can lead to the loss of your lifted butt, so be careful!

Unbeknownst to some, having a big bum is actually healthy for a woman. Carrying weight in your back as opposed to your front is much better for your posture. Also, if you have a muscular booty it can boost your metabolism, which can help you burn fat and loose weight. Gaining muscle anywhere on your body will boost your metabolism, but why not gain that muscle in an area that's both easy to target and sexy?

Health, fitness and working out are things that truly excite me and bring immense joy to my life. I love sharing my passions with others and writing is my preferred avenue for conveying my knowledge and expertise. I have a strict daily routine that I always follow and if that routine is ever broken, my body reacts negatively. The routine consists of clean eating, various forms of exercise and stretching. Many of the workouts featured in the 6-week schedule in this book are some of my personal favorites. I have also included some of my favorite healthy food recipes as well. Follow me as we take the journey to personal enhancement and getting the ass that we've always dreamed of. After reading this book you will no longer look enviously at women with lifted toned bums, rather, you will respect and understand the effort they have put into achieving it, because you will have done the same.

Fit Tip # 1:

We all have our own personal favorite comfort food and there is absolutely nothing wrong with that. But the thing about comfort foods is that the name often implies obscenely unhealthy foods. But what if we could hack our brain and alter our comfort foods to something a little more comfortable (comfortable in the sense that your body wont go into sugar shock and you wont have a ton of regret after consumption). That's right, it's possible, I should know because I've done it myself, here's how:

If you're craving something salty and crunchy, you should make some good old-fashioned popcorn. I'm not talking about the disgustingly buttery movie theatre and microwave popcorn; I'm talking about the classic stuff.

-Buy a bag of kernels

-Heat up a pot on the stove with some coconut oil in it (just a bit to avoid sticking)

-Throw in a handful of kernels and place a top over the pot

-Once you hear the first kernel pop, begin shaking the pot up a bit, ensuring that you don't lift it too far away from the heat source

-When the popping has dwindled, remove the pot from the stove and put the popcorn in a bowl

-If you want you can microwave a little bit of coconut oil and drizzle it on top

-Now you've got some options as far as what you want to put on the popcorn

Option 1- Pink Himalayan salt

Option 2- Cinnamon

Option 3- Vinegar

Option 4- Microwave a small amount of natural peanut butter and drizzle it over the popcorn

Option 5- Pink Himalayan salt, Cinnamon and a small amount of peanut butter (My personal favorite)

If popcorn just isn't doing the trick for you and you feel like you need something with a little more substance, try some natural dark chocolate. Yes you heard me right, chocolate. Dark chocolate is in a league of its own. It's packed with antioxidants; it can improve blood flow/ lower blood pressure and it can lower the risk of cardiovascular disease! I was as surprised as you probably are and I immediately made dark chocolate my go to comfort food. Dark chocolate, like anything, should obviously be consumed in moderation. The fact that eating some dark chocolate from time to time is better than stuffing your face with Reese's Pieces twice a week does not mean you should eat it all the time and abuse the positive aspects of this great comfort food. Eat it wisely!

Dieting Advice and Healthy Recipes:

As you are probably already aware, diet is arguably the most IMPORTANT FACTOR when it comes to your physical appearance. I don't care if you workout three times a day, if you are eating McDonalds and drinking Pepsi every chance you get, you will never have the body of your dreams, let alone the ass. Women naturally store more fat around their hips and bums due to a little thing called childbirth. This means that if you are eating like crap most of that crap is going to go directly to.... any guesses? If you guessed your feet, you're wrong.

If you eat like crap your lower body is going to pay the price. This means that if we want the ass of our dreams we're going to have to make some sacrifices. I know as well as anyone, sacrifices suck in the present moment, but they sure do make the final achievement taste that much sweeter. Adversity tends to build character and this scenario is no different. Gone are the days of eating whatever the hell you want, it's time to show some discipline and focus on your end goals. All the temptations that you experience are merely distractions. Discipline will allow you to tell the difference between what you want right now and what you truly desire in the future.

I will now present you with various recipes that will better allow you to prepare healthy meals. Remember, the best way to ruin a workout is to unjustifiably reward yourself with some kind of fatty snack. If you really want to feel amazing use your exercise as a motivator to continue the trend of healthy living throughout the rest of your day. Don't waste your workouts!

Blueberry Booster Smoothie:

In a blender, blend the following ingredients to your desired consistency:

1 frozen banana

1 cup of frozen blueberries

1 tbsp of flaxseed

1 tbsp of natural peanut butter

1 tsp of coconut oil

1 tsp of chia seeds

1 handful of spinach

1 handful of kale

1 cup of coconut water

1 and ½ cups of unsweetened vanilla almond milk

Sprinkle cinnamon as you desire

Notes- this smoothie packs a nutritional punch and the best part about it is that it tastes amazing. Drink this first thing in the morning and you will wake up in a hurry. It's got everything you need, protein, fiber, essential oils, fantastic hydration and amazing taste. You will not be disappointed when you try it.

Touch of Tropics Smoothie:

In a blender, blend the following ingredients to your desired consistency:

1 cup of frozen mango pieces

1 cup of strawberries

4 dates

1 tbsp of natural almond butter

2 rings of pineapple (sliced up)

1 tsp of coconut oil

1 tsp of chia seeds

1 cup of coconut water

1 and ½ cups of unsweetened vanilla almond milk

Notes- this smoothie is simply delicious and it will energize you like nothing else. If you want to make the consistency a bit more liquid you can add an extra ½ cup of coconut water.

Green Beast Smoothie:

In a blender, blend the following ingredients to your desired consistency:

2 cups of kale

1 cup of spinach

1 tbsp of natural peanut butter

2 dates

1 stalk of celery

½ of an avocado

2 cups of coconut water

¼ cup of almond milk

Notes- you may find that the taste of this smoothie isn't quite on par with the previous two, but the nutritional value of the ingredients cannot be overlooked. Sacrificing taste for nutrition isn't always a bad thing.

Quinoa Breakfast Beauty:

1 cup of quinoa

2 cups of water

1 tsp of cinnamon

¼ cup of dried cranberries

1 tsp of sliced almonds

¼ cup of almond milk

drizzle almond butter as desired

Notes- boil 1 cup of quinoa in 2 cups of water until all the water has been absorbed and the quinoa is no longer hard. Serve yourself a bowl (put the leftovers in the fridge). After you have your bowl you can then put the rest of the ingredients on to add flavor. This is a simple and hearty breakfast that is a fantastic alternative to oatmeal.

Kale & Spinach Super Salad:

In a bowl mix the following ingredients.

A generous amount of kale and spinach

1 tsp of Pumpkin seeds

1 tsp of Chia seeds

1 tsp of ground flaxseeds

1 avocado

¼ cup of chickpeas

¼ cup of black beans

Drizzle balsamic vinegar and canola oil as desired for dressing

Notes- if you don't like the taste of the balsamic dressing you can use something else. Try to go for something low in fat though.

The Tuna Treat:

Ingredients

1 can of tuna

Cherry tomatoes

1 avocado

1 tsp of coconut oil

1 Mango

Open the can of tuna, heat up 1 tsp of coconut oil in a frying pan and lightly cook the tuna of 1-2 minutes. Slice up your avocado, cherry tomatoes and mango. Put the cooked tuna in a bowl with the avocado and tomatoes. I like to drizzle siracha sauce and honey over the meal and mix it up with a fork before eating. The taste of hot and sweet from the honey and siracha sauce is delectable!

Let's be honest here, deep down we all know when we are eating bad foods. We know the difference between healthy and unhealthy eating no matter how many times we may try to make justifications in our minds. Human beings are very good at rationalization, but you need to completely eliminate the idea of bad food rationalization from your psyche. While a cheat day once a week or a couple cheat meals throughout the week are perfectly fine and actually recommended, consistently eating crappy foods day after day and trying to justify it by snacking on celery and salad is not a good idea. If you want that nice shapely booty you need to make some sacrifices and it all starts with your diet!

Fit Tip # 2:

This is the easiest tip to start implementing immediately. Once I started doing this I found it a lot easier to get myself out of bed in the morning and begin my workout.

Put your alarm clock as far away as you can from your bed, whether it be an actual alarm clock, your phone, watch, or whatever device you use to wake up the morning. Make sure your alarm is on full volume so that there is no chance of you ignoring it. By forcing yourself to hop up out of bed and walk over to turn your alarm clock off, it will decrease your chances of crawling back into bed for another "5 minutes" of sleep that can often turn into 45.

If you put your alarm clock within arms reach like most people do, you don't have to exert any effort to turn it off. But by getting up out of bed to turn it off you have to make the conscious choice of getting back into your bed, even though you know you should just stay standing because you've already got the hardest part of waking up out of the way.

If you really want you can actually put your alarm outside of your room, if you're confident in the fact that your alarm is loud enough to hear from a distance. Whichever method you decide to do, make sure you start doing it right away because it will make your morning a whole lot easier!

Explanation of Key Exercises:

Here I will be explaining all of the exercises that you will have to do in the 6-week program. I will do my best to explain them all but if any of them seem unclear there are certainly YouTube videos out there that can give you a more in-depth idea on how to do particular exercises.

Understanding Workout Terminology:

When reading a workout the first number is the number of sets and the second number is the number of repetitions per set. So if you see 4 x 20, that means four sets of twenty reps per set. During a set you perform every exercise in order with no rest between exercises unless otherwise instructed. Some workouts will be timed such as 3 x 1:00, 1:00 off, 1:30 on. For this workout you would be doing each exercise in the set for one minute, resting for one minute and then doing that same exercise for one and a half minutes.

The Kettle Bell Swing:

You can use dumbbells instead of kettle bells; it's just a little harder to hold onto them. Remember to start light, grip the kettle bell with two hands, let it swing between your legs, slightly bend your knees, then thrust your hips and straighten your legs simultaneously while keeping your back straight to swing the kettle bell up to eye level. Arms should be slightly bent, feet at shoulder width apart. The weight you use is totally dependent on the number of repetitions you will be doing. If you are a beginner I recommend starting with 20-25 lbs. Your arms should not be doing much work at all, they are simply holding and guiding the kettle bell, the power of your swing should be coming from your legs, hips, core and back.

The Burpee:

Start in the standing position, jump down until your chest is on the ground, do a pushup keeping your back flat, jump your legs up into a squatted position and spring yourself up into the air with your arms reaching to the sky. With practice this movement will become fluid, but it remains a very challenging exercise.

The Squat:

Squats should be performed with your feet at shoulder width apart. Put your arms straight out in front of you and keep your back straight as you lower your bum to your ankles, keeping your legs parallel to one-another. Keep your back straight and keep your weight on your heels. Once you get as low as you can, use your legs to push yourself back up to the standing position, all the while keeping your back straight and your core tight. Some workouts require weighted squats, I recommend holding a dumbbell in each of your hands, with your arms straight when performing weighted squats.

The Mountain Climber:

Mountain climbers are great for your core. To perform, hover above the ground keeping your body horizontal. You should be on your toes and hands with your arms straight. One at a time, bring your knees towards your chest in an alternating motion. Every time both legs go in and out, you have completed one repetition.

Squat Jumps:

Squat jumps are performed just like a regular squat, but you jump into the air about 1 foot upon extension of the legs.

The Plank:

For a plank you want your stomach facing the ground. Put your elbows underneath your shoulders and lift yourself off the ground. Your weight should be on your elbows and your toes. Try to keep your back perfectly flat (don't sag your hips down to the ground or lift your bum really high into the air). Keep your abs tight and ensure that you have a comfortable base on your elbows/ forearms.

Leg Ins:

Leg ins are done from the plank position. Once in position, bring your right knee to your right elbow, and then back. Do the same with your left side and that equates to two reps.

Pikes:

 Pikes are also done from the plank position. Simply arch your back and stick your bum into the air, returning to the plank position to complete one repetition.

The Lunge Walk:

One leg at a time, step one foot out in front of you as far as you can, while dropping the opposite knee down to the ground (don't actually touch the knee on the ground, but get as close as you can). Get a nice smooth walking pattern going as you continue to switch legs.

Wall Sits:

Put your back flat against a wall, bend your legs at about 90 degrees and hover above the ground like you are sitting in an invisible chair. Hold the position for as long as the specified time says.

Leg Ups:

 While holding onto a pull-up bar with your arms straight, bring your knees up to your chest and flex your abs.

Plank Leg Lifts:

From the basic plank position alternately lift your legs up into the air. Lift both legs once to complete one rep

Speed Skaters:

Swing your left leg behind you (in a sort of sideways lunge) and touch your right foot with your right hand, then swing your right leg behind you and touch your left foot with your left hand to complete one rep.

High Knees:

Run on the spot with your knees coming up to your chest. Each time both legs go up and down you've done 1 rep

Kneeling Super Mans:

Start on your hands and knees. Reach your right arm out straight in front of you and extend your left leg behind you. Once extended bring your right elbow to your left knee. Do the same with your left arm and right leg to complete one rep.

Hip Raises:

Lie flat on your back with your knees bent. Thrust your hips upwards so that your butt is off the ground and then lower your bum back onto the ground. Do this in a slow and controlled motion, keeping your glutes flexed the entire time.

Single Leg Hip Raises:

This is just like regular hip raises except you are going to do one leg at a time. When you are using your right leg to push your hips into the air, your left leg should be straight and vice-versa. You will find this more challenging but it really helps target each specific side of your bum.

Jumping Jacks:

Do I need to explain this one? Hop your legs in towards each other and then hop them out until they are past shoulder width. While jumping, your straight arms should be simultaneously following the motion of your legs. Essentially when your legs come together, your arms are at your side, when you jump your legs apart your arms swing up towards the sky so that your whole body looks like a star.

Squat Walk:

From the squat position, hold your arms straight out in front of you and walk to one side. Face forward and don't cross your feet. Step out to the side with one foot and follow with your other. Each step is one repetition. Try to walk in each direction for an equal number of repetitions.

6-Week Training Schedule:

Week 1:
MONDAY:

 1 set of:

30 high knees

20 kettle bell swings

20 kneeling superman's

30 jumping jacks

20 mountain climbers

10 burpees

30 jumping jacks

20 squats

30 lunge walks

30 high knees

*Rest 20 seconds between exercises.

TUESDAY:

3 sets of 45 seconds of the following exercises:

Plank

Hip Raises

Wall Sits

* Rest 1 minute between exercises and 2 minutes between sets.

NOTE: If you cant hold the exercises for 45 seconds at a time, take breaks as you need but try to resume to exercise as quickly as you can.

WEDNESDAY:

20 minute jog

THURSDAY:

10 minutes of as many sets as you can complete of:

10 squats

6 lunge Walks

3 burpees

NOTE: Keep track of how many sets you completed to gauge future progress in the same workout.

FRIDAY:

3 X 15-20 reps of the following 6 exercises

plank leg lifts

kneeling superman's

hip raises

speed skates

lunge walk

pike

*Rest 20 seconds between exercises and 2 minutes between sets

SATURDAY:

Rest Day.

Try to complete 30 minutes of stretching during your rest days. Stretching consistently will help you to strengthen yours muscles and prevent injury. Create a stretching routine that works for you and that you can complete regularly.

SUNDAY:

30 minute jog

Weekly Review:

1 week down, 5 more to go. Excellent job! This week had some of the shorter workout featured in it, so be prepared for some more volume and intensity in the coming weeks. Remember, as the workouts get more difficult to keep that diet in check. You don't want to spoil all of your hard work with a few moments of pleasure as you eat something unhealthy.

Week 2:

MONDAY:

Perform 2:00 of the exercise, rest for 45 seconds, perform 1:00 of the same exercise, and then proceed to move down the list:

Squat jumps

Lunge walks

Squat walks

Plank

Ketlle bell swings

Pikes

TUESDAY:

3 X (2:00 plank, 1:00 rest, 1:30 plank)

* Rest 4:00 between sets

WEDNESDAY:

30 minute jog

THURSDAY:

4 sets of:

25 squats

20 single leg hip raises

30 kneeling superman's

40 high knees

25 speed skaters

50 plank leg lifts

*Rest 2:30 between sets and don't rest between exercises

FRIDAY:

4 sets of:

50 kettle bell swings

30 leg ups

1:00 plank

30 mountain climbers

1:30 wall sits

40 hips raises

*Rest 2:00 between sets and 20 seconds between exercises.

SATURDAY:

Rest day

SUNDAY:

2 sets of

10 minute jog

50 squats

10 minute jog

*Rest 3 minutes between sets

Weekly Review:

Keep up the great work! The intensity of the workouts is going to continue with each week that passes. Keep your goals in mind and let's keep working towards the booty you've always dreamed of!

Fit Tip # 3:

Maintaining mobility and flexibility is a crucial aspect of fitness. Getting into simple 5-10 minute morning yoga routines can really make the difference between feeling stiff for the day, and feeling loose and mobile. There are tons of quick YouTube videos that will provide you with free yoga videos. All it takes is a few sun salutations and some of your favorite stretches/ poses.

Before I even begin my morning workout I like to do some yoga to get warmed up. Doing yoga and focused breathing before bed is also a very relaxing ritual to get into. You can even do focused breathing while lying in bed. Here's what I sometimes like to do:

- Close your eyes
- Breathe in for 5 seconds and out for 5 seconds
- Continue this breathing pattern and focus on relaxing your entire body, starting at your toes and slowly working your way up to your neck
- With every breath try focusing on relaxing a different part of your body, for examples: 5 seconds in 5 seconds out at your feet, 5 seconds in 5 seconds out at your calves, 5 seconds in 5 seconds out at your knees, etc.
- Once you have worked your way up your entire body breath in and out deeply one last time, inhaling for as long as possible and exhaling in as slow and controlled of a manner as your can.

Doing yoga first thing in the morning will definitely prepare you for a workout and doing it right before bed will help you sleep like a baby.

Week 3:

MONDAY:

10 kettle bell swings, 1 squat

9 kettle bell swings, 2 squats

8 kettle bell swings, 3 squats

7 kettle bell swings, 4 squats

6 kettle bell swings, 5 squats

5 kettle bell swings, 6 squats

4 kettle bell swings, 7 squats

3 kettle bell swings, 8 squats

2 kettle bell swings, 9 squats

1 kettle bell swing, 10 squats

REST for 1 minute

10 squats, 1 kettle bell swing

9 squats, 2 kettle bell swings

8 squats, 3 kettle bell swings

7 squats, 4 kettle bell swings

6 squats, 5 kettle bell swings

5 squats, 6 kettle bell swings

4 squats, 7 kettle bell swings

3 squats, 8 kettle bell swings

2 squats, 9 kettle bell swings

1 squat, 10 kettle bell swings

TUESDAY:

10 minutes of as many sets as you can complete of:

10 squats

6 lunge Walks

3 burpees

NOTE: Write down your result and compare the results of this workout to the previous one you completed in week 1.

WEDNESDAY:

6 sets of 10-12 reps of the following exercises:

squats (weighted)

burpees

single leg hip raises

leg ups

mountain climbers

speed skaters

THURSDAY:

45 minute jog

FRIDAY:

Rest day

SATURDAY:

Run for 20 minutes then perform 3 sets of the following:

1:00 kettle bell swings

30 seconds of pikes

1:00 high knees

30 seconds squat jumps

1:00 plank leg lifts

30 seconds burpees

*Rest 2:00 between sets, no rest between exercises.

SUNDAY:

6 X jog for 3:00, sprint for 1:00, perform burpees for 1:00

*Rest for 2:00 between sets and do not rest between exercises. On the rest you should be walking, not stationary.

Weekly Review:

That was a tough week and if you've made it to this point without missing a single workout, congratulations! You need to be focusing on your eating habits just as much as you focus on the workout schedule. Keep it up!

Week 4:

MONDAY:

Do as many sets as possible in twenty minutes, rest as needed.

10 squat jumps

10 burpees

10 kettle bell swings

10 kneeling superman's

10 hip raises

10 pikes

TUESDAY:

2 sets of:

50 squats

40 hip raises

30 squat walks

20 plank leg lifts

10 squat jumps

5 burpees

*Rest 3 minutes between sets and do not rest between exercises

WEDNESDAY:

Rest day

THURSDAY:

1 hour jog

* Rest as needed. but try to run for the entire 1-hour duration. If you must rest do not stop, simply walk until you are able to run again.

FRIDAY:

1 set of:

1:00 wall sit

1:00 plank

1:00 squat walk

Rest for 2 minutes

1:30 wall sit

1:30 plank

1:30 squat walk

Rest for 2 minutes

2:00 wall sit

2:00 plank

2:00 squat walk

NOTES: This is a challenging workout. For the squat walks simply perform repetitions until the time is up. Having a stopwatch is a good idea for this workout.

SATURDAY:

Total 40 minutes of running. During the 40 minutes you will stop every 5 minutes and perform 15 squats, 10 lunge walks and 3 burpees.

Make sure you stop your watch timer while you're doing your exercise set and be sure to resume the watch timer when you begin running again.

SUNDAY:

6 sets of:

20 lunge walks

10 high knees

20 squat jumps

10 jumping jacks

20 kettle bell swings

10 high knees

20 plank leg lifts

10 jumping jacks

*Rest 30 seconds between exercises and 2 minutes between sets

Weekly Review:

As the weeks get tougher, so do you! Hopefully at this point you are starting to feel and see you bum tightening up and lifting. Looking in the mirror and seeing results is one of the most satisfying feelings you can have, so enjoy it, you've earned it.

Fit Tip # 4

I could have made this book very simple by saying:

"If you want a nice, lifted ass, do the following while mainlining a healthy diet:"

Day 1- 10 squats

Day 2- 20 squats

Day 3- 30 squats

Day 4- 40 squats

I think you see the trend, but what's the problem with this you ask? Repetition does not give you results. The following is a quote that I think is applicable:

"Never give your body a simple solution or let it get comfortable. Always keep your body guessing so it's able to do what it does best, adapt to the most adverse and arduous of circumstances.

-John Mayo

Doing the same workout here and there isn't necessarily a bad thing, but if you do the same exercise routine day after day your body is going to hit a progress plateau and you will stop seeing results. You must constantly vary your workouts and that is exactly what you will be doing if you follow this 6-week program.

Week 5:

MONDAY:

5 x 30 reps of:

kettle bell swings

squat jumps

mountain climbers

lunge walks

*Rest 2:00 between sets and don't rest between exercises

TUESDAY:

Jog for 20 minutes and then do:

4 sets of

Max duration hip raise

Max duration plank

Max duration wall sit

*Rest for 1 minute between exercises and 2 minutes between sets.

NOTES: For this workout you are simply holding the given exercise pose for as long as you possibly can. For hip raises, instead of doing repetitions you are going to lift your hips off of the ground and hold the position for as long as possible. Keep track of how long you're doing each exercise and try to remain as consistent as possible as you complete the 4 sets.

WEDNESDAY:

Each main exercise is accompanied by an easier, alternate exercise. Perform 1:00 of the main exercise and 1:30 of the alternate exercise. On the second set perform 1:30 of the main exercise and 1:00 of the alternate exercise.

Perform 2 sets of the following:

main: squats, alt: jumping jacks

main: burpees, alt: plank leg lifts

main: leg ins, alt: high knees

main: lunge walks, alt: rest

main: kettle bell swings, alt: leg ups

main: kneeling superman's, alt: hip raises

*Rest 30 seconds between exercises and 6 minutes between sets. Do not rest while transitioning from the main exercise to the alternate exercise.

THURSDAY:

1-hour jog/walk broken down as follows:

6 Sets of:

walk for 2 minutes

jog for 6 minutes

sprint for 1 minute

walk for 1 minute

*No rest, the walking portion should be enough rest for this workout.

FRIDAY:

Rest day

SATURDAY:

Perform sets 1, 2, 3 and after resting for 5 minutes perform sets 3, 2, 1.

Set 1:

20 seconds of each of the following exercises

Burpees

Squat walks

Mountain climbers

Pikes

Set 2:

30 seconds of each of the following exercises

Kneeling superman's

Plank leg lifts

Lunge walks

Speed skaters

Set 3:

45 seconds of each of the following exercises

Leg ups

Kettle bell swings

Leg ins

Hip raises

*Rest 10 seconds between exercises and 1:30 between sets. Rest 5 minutes after completing sets 1, 2 and 3.

NOTES: In total you will be completing each set two times.

SUNDAY:

40 minute jog

Every 10 minutes stop your watch and perform 20 squat jumps, 20 lunge walks and 30 high knees

*No rest

Weekly Review:

You just completed your second last week of the training program, excellent work! Next week will be just as challenging as this one, but it's the final week so let's get it done!

Week 6:

MONDAY:

3 sets of:

40 high knees

30 kettle bell swings

20 kneeling superman's

40 jumping jacks

20 mountain climbers

10 burpees

40 jumping jacks

20 squats

30 lunge walks

30 high knees

*Rest 20 seconds between exercises and 2 minutes between sets

TUESDAY:

40 minute jog

WEDNESDAY:

Rest day

THURSDAY:

20-minute jog, rest for 10 minutes and then do:

10 minutes of as many sets as you can complete of:

10 squats

6 lunge Walks

3 burpees

NOTE: Write down your result and compare the results of this workout to the previous ones you completed in week 1 and week 3.

FRIDAY:

You have 25 minutes to gather as many points as possible. I suggest doing this with a friend and seeing who can get the most points. The harder the exercise, the more points it's worth.

Jumping jacks- 1pt

High knees- 1pt

Hip raises- 1pt

Mountain climbers- 2pts

Kneeling superman's- 2pts

Speed skaters- 2pts

Plank- 3pts for every 5 seconds

Leg ups- 3pts

Pikes- 3pts

Squats- 4pts

Plank leg lifts- 4 pts

Lunge walks- 4pts

Wall sits- 5pts for every 10 seconds

Burpees- 5pts

Squat Jumps- 5pts

SATURDAY:

Jog a total of 1 hour, broken down as follows:

12 sets of:

Jog for 4:30, Sprint for 30 seconds

*No rest, continue jogging directly after you are finished sprinting.

SUNDAY:

6 sets of the following:

40 hip raises

50 kneeling superman's

30 leg ups

2 minutes plank

30 leg ins

50 jumping jacks

30 plank leg lifts

50 squats

*Rest 20 seconds between exercises and 3 minutes between sets

Weekly Review:

Congratulations, you have successfully completed the 6-week training program and hopefully you have noticed some great results. Having a nice bum doesn't stop here; you need to maintain your figure. You now have a myriad of different workouts at your disposal that you can regularly do to maintain the ass of your dreams.

Conclusion:

I hope you have found this book useful, informative and fun. I will be releasing more books in the near future, all of which will help you live a healthier, fitter and more fulfilling life. Never give up on your fitness goals and always continue to move forward. The main thing that I hope you learned from this book is how to hold yourself accountable for your own fitness. As a personal trainer, I'm aware of how expensive hiring a trainer can be and obviously not everybody can afford the luxury of having someone directly guide them to a greater fitness level. This is why I love writing, because I can provide cheap workout content for those people that truly need to.

If you want to live a healthy life you must rely on yourself and nobody else. If you don't truly desire to be more fit, then it doesn't matter how many personal trainers you have. I've had clients who swear to me that they want to lose weight, gain muscle, get abs, tone their butt, or whatever the case may be. But the point is that words will only get you so far, you must take action, which is exactly what you've done by reading this book, congratulations!

If you enjoyed this book I would ask that you please leave a review, it would be greatly appreciated.